52-WEEK MINDFULNESS PLANNER

A Year of Daily Inspiration & Joyful Journaling

ANNE MARIE O'CONNOR

CENTENNIAL BOOKS

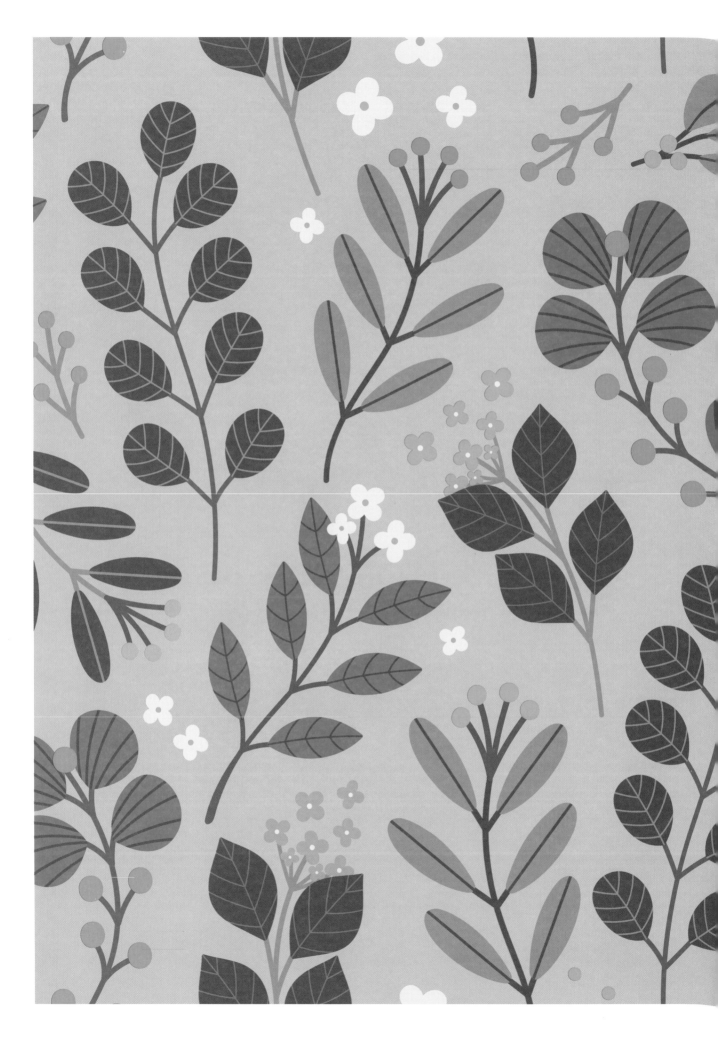

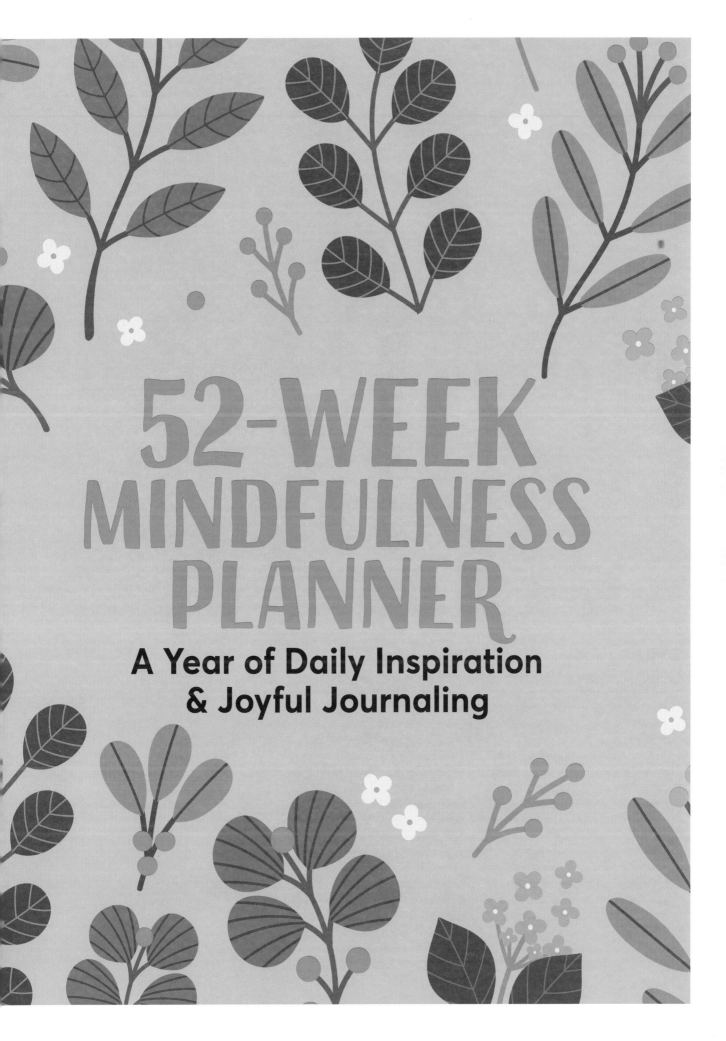

52-WEEK MINDFULNESS PLANNER

A Year of Daily Inspiration & Joyful Journaling

MAKING *NEW* NEW YEAR'S RESOLUTIONS

When it comes to setting your goals for 2022—
and actually keeping them—mindfulness is
the secret to long-term sustainability.
Here's how to set yourself up for success.

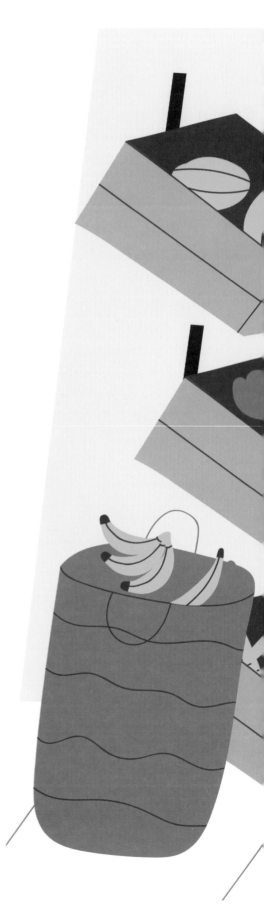

You've undoubtedly heard—or just as likely experienced firsthand—that New Year's resolutions don't stick, at least not for most of us. I won't bore you with statistics, but the number of people who manage to stay committed to their lofty January 1 goals is gloomy at best. What starts off as a shiny new blueprint for finally getting that body you've always wanted (keto! intermittent fasting!), saving loads of money (Starbucks, *moi*?) or knitting a whole new wardrobe, can lose momentum even before that shipment of expensive low-carb ketchup you ordered from Amazon arrives on your doorstep.

Which is why I've always forgone resolutions altogether. Why make some unrealistic (albeit well-intentioned) promise that I won't be able to keep, solely in the name of the New Year (and OK, probably to help counter too much holiday indulgence)?

Well, it turns out I might be missing out. "The new year *can* be a good catalyst for trying new things or dropping old habits," says Bryan Aston, LMSW, the director of training at Mindful Psychotherapy Services in New York City. But before you resolve to swear off sugar or compete in a marathon, there's something you should do first: "Ask yourself questions like, why am I doing this, and why am I doing this right now? It's about having awareness that it's not just about the goal, such as stopping smoking or overeating; it's about the triggers that

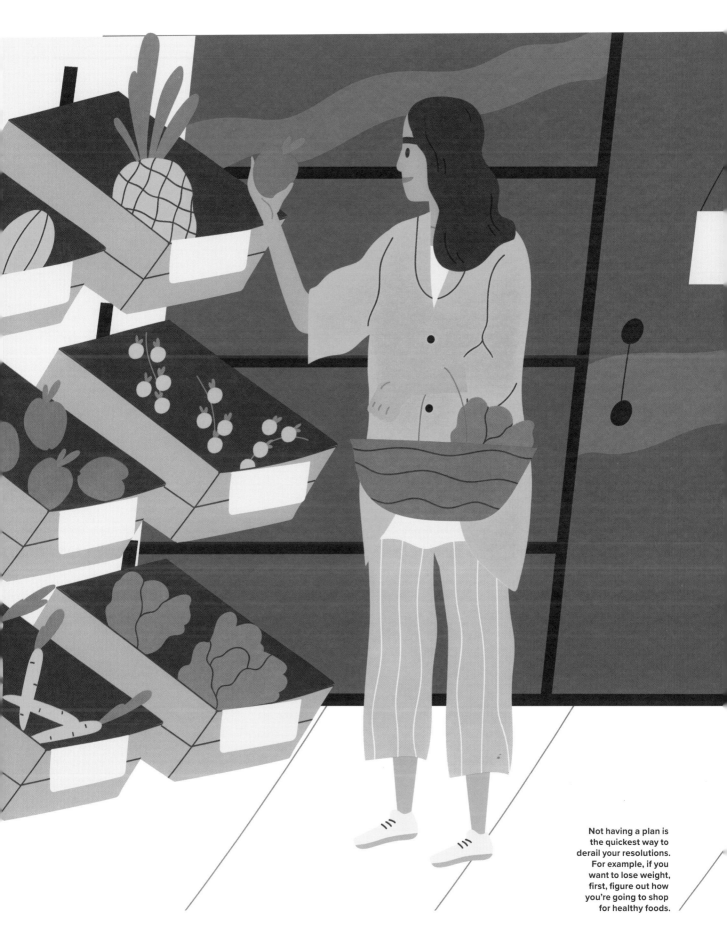

Not having a plan is the quickest way to derail your resolutions. For example, if you want to lose weight, first, figure out how you're going to shop for healthy foods.

make you reach for that cigarette or that extra cookie. What are you going to do in those times instead?"

In other words, sticking to your resolutions requires a closer examination of the situations you regularly find yourself in. Being more mindful is the key to seeing the bigger picture, which will help you make real, lasting changes that have the power to impact your overall well-being. Here's how to harness the powers of awareness and being in the moment to create a road map for resolution success—because there's no time better than the present.

BEFORE YOU MAKE A RESOLUTION...

THINK IT THROUGH

It can be tempting to want to go full steam ahead with your goal the moment January 1 comes around. But "it's important to know that just because you set a resolution doesn't mean you have to start it right away," Aston says. "You can think about it, and really put the measures into place to set yourself up for success."

To wit: We've all known people (or been that person) who signed up for a gym membership right at the start of the year. In hopes of losing weight fast, they resolve to go to class five days a week, but quickly get bored or injured. A more mindful approach would be researching fitness options nearby and finding one with classes that suit both your schedule and your interests—even if that means not starting until February 1. (Bonus: It will be much less crowded.)

BE THE SNAIL

New Year's resolutions that fail share a common denominator. "People tend to set a lot of expectations in terms of breaking a habit that they've

Mindful movement— yoga, tai chi, qi gong— can help you stay focused on your goals.

most likely had for a very long time," Aston says. So instead of going cold turkey, he advocates going for harm reduction. "This approach is about taking baby steps and making small, incremental changes."

For example, "let's say you're trying to quit smoking, which is a very difficult habit to break. Maybe you'll start by saying that you're only going to smoke at designated times each day or you'll smoke only half a cigarette at a time." Once you're successful with this mini goal, then you can move onto the next goal (smoking fewer times a day or only taking three puffs), and then the next, until you've fulfilled your ultimate goal.

HAVE SOME (SELF) COMPASSION

When setting your goal, don't lose sight of your present situation. "Ask yourself, what can I handle at this time?" Aston advises. "If you have three kids, a partner and a job, is going to the gym five times per week something you can really stick to?"

If the answer is no, find a happy medium, which is something that feels more comfortable—and that you'll be more likely to sustain. "Give yourself a bit more leniency. Simply deciding that you want to begin a new habit is something that should be applauded. In this case, that might be starting with just a Saturday workout class," says Aston.

AFTER YOU MAKE YOUR RESOLUTION...

DON'T *JUST* HOLD YOURSELF ACCOUNTABLE

Perhaps as important as making a commitment to your own goals is finding someone to help you stay committed, Aston says. Besides planning how you're going to accomplish the goal, it's also essential to enlist someone who can help you stick with it. "We need someone external to keep us on track," he explains. "People are more likely to

follow through if they know they're being held accountable."

If your goal is, say, starting a regular workout regimen, a personal trainer is the ideal person to keep you in check. "You get individualized attention *and* accountability," says Aston.

If you can't afford a trainer, try the buddy system. "If you have a friend who also wants to get in shape, make a date with them to go walking each week," suggests Aston.

> "AVOID JUDGMENTAL LANGUAGE," SAYS BRYAN ASTON, LMSW. "IF YOU HAVE A SLICE OF CAKE, DON'T THINK, 'I'M OFF THE WAGON.' IT JUST MEANS YOU HAD A SLICE OF CAKE."

HONE YOUR AWARENESS SKILLS

To stay on track with your resolution, Aston says it's imperative to learn to manage your daily stressors as they come up. "Say something stressful arises at work and you want to go for a cigarette break. That ability to recognize what it is that causes you to reach for that cigarette in the first place—that external thought and the feeling that comes on, such as anxiety, sadness or even boredom—is necessary before you can restructure it. Once you're able to do that, you can replace it with another thought or a distraction."

Finding something that can disrupt these behaviors, especially when it comes to super-ingrained habits like smoking and overeating, can be a process of trial and error, Aston says. "It probably won't work on

that first try, but there is a method that will work." (See below for some mindfulness tools to help you.)

Also, if you do slip, don't just abandon your goal; instead, take a moment to think about what triggered you and how you can avoid it in the future.

BUILD YOUR MINDFULNESS TOOLBOX

Stay focused on the bigger picture with these techniques from Bryan Aston, LMSW:

1 **Wear a brightly colored bracelet or rubber band.** "Pull it or snap it to help bring you back to the present moment."

2 **Get out of there.** "Remove yourself from whatever it is that's triggering you. So if you're in the break room and see a big, gorgeous chocolate cake and you know that might be a trigger, remove yourself from that situation"—for example, by taking a walk.

3 **Breathe through your nose.** "Breathing slowly and deeply through your nose is best when we want to engage our executive functioning, which is what allows us to have more rational thoughts. Breathing through the mouth, on the other hand, can mimic hyperventilation."

4 **Put pen to paper.** "For weight loss, especially, journaling can be effective. Instead of writing down how many calories you eat, which can be very shaming, write down everything you ate that day (and not just each meal). Also, jot down the experience you had with it—e.g., the cookie at work made you feel guilty. It's not meant to be shameful; it's meant to promote awareness."

5 **Engage in mindful movement.** Texting on the treadmill is the equivalent of watching TV while you devour dinner. Instead, focus on what you're doing. "Activities that combine breath with movement, like qi gong, are most effective," Aston says. Pilates and yoga are other good options. —*Amanda Altman*

THE BENEFITS OF MINDFULNESS

Nothing gives you a bigger bang for your buck than practices like meditation, journaling and yoga.

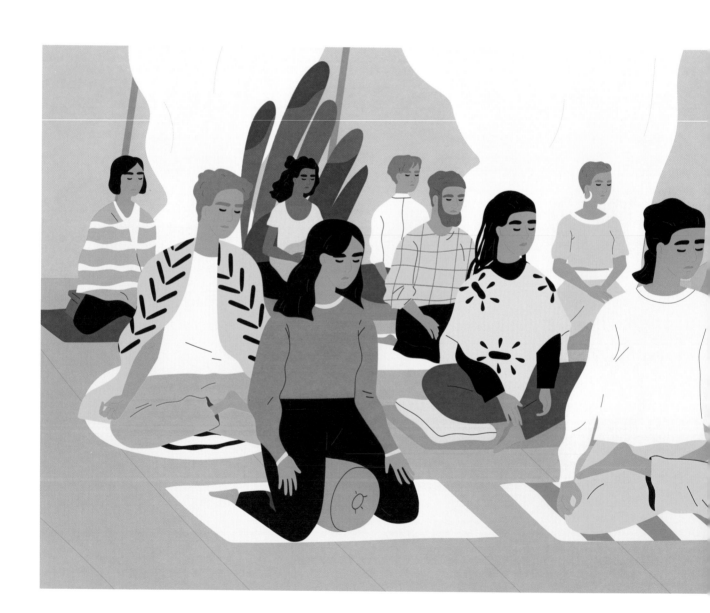

Imagine how it would feel if, by the end of this year, you felt less stressed and anxious, more focused and more content. And, as an added benefit, your physical health was improved. Bonus: It doesn't require huge expenditures or marathon-training-level efforts, and you can do it pretty much anywhere. And it doesn't require tons of time.

SO WHAT IS THIS "WONDER DRUG"?

Research shows that mindfulnesss might very well indeed be the Holy Grail when it comes to both physical and emotional well-being. It's generally defined as the act of being aware of what you're sensing and feeling in the moment, so that you can direct your attention away from negative thoughts and worries. "The really exciting thing about practicing mindfulness is we now have the modern diagnostic tools to understand how this thousands-of-years-old tradition truly affects the mind and body," explains Ben Karlin, a meditation instructor and founder of Free Form Minds, a company that works with employers to cultivate mindfulness within their workplace.

The good news is mindfulness is a quality all of us possess: "You just have to learn the tools to access it," says Karlin. Even better, you can do it in short bursts throughout the day, or nurture it through other mediums like journaling or yoga. There are many ways to practice mindfulness, and in ways that are easy and doable even in today's hectic, fast-paced, changing 24/7 world.

HERE ARE SOME OF THE REASONS YOU SHOULD TRY MINDFULNESS...

IT IMPROVES DEPRESSION AND ANXIETY

A 2014 *JAMA* review of 47 trials involving over 3,500 participants suggests that mindfulness-meditation programs help improve both anxiety

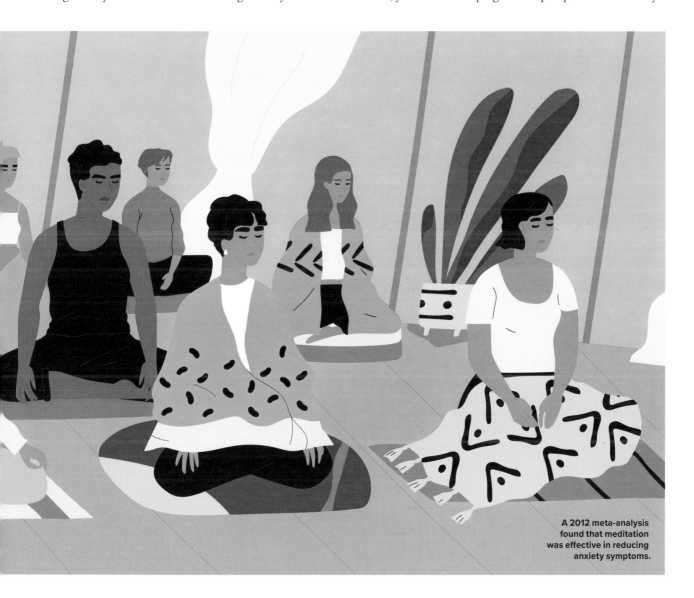

A 2012 meta-analysis found that meditation was effective in reducing anxiety symptoms.

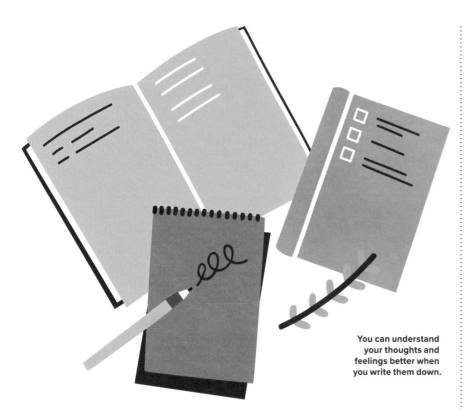

You can understand your thoughts and feelings better when you write them down.

meditation appears to lower heart rate and blood pressure, according to a 2018 Michigan Technological University study.

IT LOWERS YOUR CHANCES OF DEVELOPING DEMENTIA

One UCLA study published in 2016 in the *Journal of Alzheimer's Disease* found that people over the age of 55 who took a one-hour weekly meditative yoga class and meditated at home for 12 minutes a day for three months had significant improvements in verbal memory (remembering word lists) and visual-spatial memory (the ability to find and remember locations). These practices "help reduce stress and inflammation, which are both toxic to the brain," explains Englehart. They may also help enhance production of brain-derived neurotrophic growth factor (BDNF)—a protein that stimulates connections between your brain neurons.

IT BOOSTS YOUR IMMUNE SYSTEM

When you're stressed, inflammation in your body increases. That in turn can lower levels of infection-fighting cells in your body, so you're more susceptible to colds and flu. But

and depression. Another 2016 review published in *JAMA Psychiatry* found that mindfulness-based cognitive therapy was just as effective as antidepressants in preventing depression relapses in patients. "One reason is that mindfulness allows people to be more intentionally aware of the present moment, which helps them step back to understand their own reactions and avoid getting swept up in negative emotions like sadness or anger," explains Jessica Englehart, LPCC-S, ATR, RYT, a senior clinical consultant in the mindfulness program at OhioHealth Behavioral Health Outpatient Services in Columbus, Ohio. Being in the moment allows you to savor life's pleasures and be fully engaged in the moment, and it gives you a greater capacity to deal with stress and negative events.

IT REDUCES YOUR RISK OF HEART DISEASE

A 2013 study published in the journal *Psychosomatic Medicine* found

that people with prehypertension (high blood pressure) who practiced mindfulness techniques for 2.5 hours a week for eight weeks had significantly greater reductions in their blood pressure than those who didn't. You don't have to do much to see effects, either: Just one hour of

By focusing exclusively on the process of drinking a cup of tea, Zen Buddhist monks have turned it into a form of meditation.

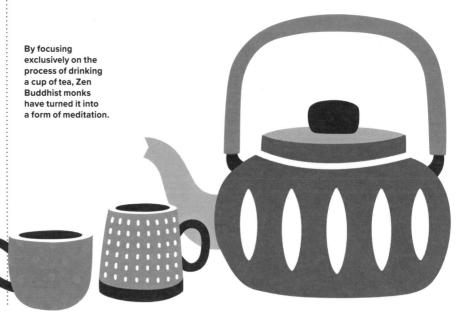

mindfulness can offset that: A 2012 study of adults over the age of 50 who participated in an eight-week mindfulness-based stress reduction (MBSR) program found that they had fewer sick days and less severe symptoms when they did fall ill than a control group.

A SIMPLE MINDFULNESS PRACTICE

"What I tell people is, finding small but daily ways to practice is a good way to get started—squeezing in just five minutes once a day is better than a half-hour once a week, because daily practice helps reset your brain's neural circuitry," explains Karlin. Start with this short practice:

- ✔ Sit in a spot that feels calm and quiet.
- ✔ Set a time limit of 5 to 10 minutes.
- ✔ Notice your body. Whether you're sitting on a chair or cross-legged on a floor, lying down or kneeling, make sure that it's a position that is stable and comfortable.
- ✔ Focus on your breath. Breathe like you normally would, in and out of your nose. Your eyes can be open or closed.
- ✔ If your mind wanders, it's OK— just try to bring attention back to your breath. Over time, you'll notice that it becomes less and less frequent as you strengthen your practice. "It's common for your mind to drift off to something else— it's impossible to keep your thoughts, sleepiness or anxiety at bay," says Alice Domar, PhD, executive director of the Domar Center for Mind/Body Health in Massachusetts.

Once you've gotten into a consistent schedule of practicing mindfulness every day, you can step it up a notch, building up to 10, 20, even 30 minutes with practice. There's also no set rule that you have to do it for a set amount of time. "Three minutes of meditating while waiting in the carpool line is great—you'll still get benefits," says Domar. In fact, squeezing even just a bit of mindfulness practice in when you can is a great strategy when you're strapped for time.

You can also practice mindfulness in other forms, like tai chi or yoga. A relatively new form of yoga called Mindful Yoga, for example, applies traditional mindfulness techniques to yoga moves like the standard tree or mountain pose. "By having you really focus on your breath as you do the various poses, it encourages your mind to become more in tune with your body," says Englehart. "It also promotes more body awareness, which in turn encourages us to take care of the only bodies we're given."

GIVING THANKS

Another option is keeping a gratitude journal, where you write down up to five things that you feel grateful for every day. One study published in the *Journal of Personality and Social Psychology* found that people who kept one for two weeks experienced more gratitude, positive moods and optimism about the future than a control group. "At the end of the day, the best type of mindfulness practice for you is the one you're most likely to stick to, whatever its form," says Englehart.

—*Hallie Levine*

HOW TO CHOOSE THE BEST MEDITATION STYLE FOR YOU

It's not a one-size-fits-all practice.
Find the type that suits you.

→ MINDFULNESS MEDITATION
This type of meditation really forces you to focus on the sights, sounds and smells around you that ordinarily slip on by.
Best for people who want to increase their ability to focus and ignore distractions and become more resilient under stress.

→ BREATH AWARENESS MEDITATION
This technique, also known as mindful breathing, focuses your attention on your breath, both the inhale and exhale.
Best for beginners just learning the ropes.

→ TRANSCENDENTAL MEDITATION
Often also known as mantra meditation, this type of meditation uses a repetitive sound, like "om," to clear the mind.

Best for people who find it hard to focus just on their breath, or are uncomfortable with silence.

→ LOVING KINDNESS MEDITATION
Also known as "metta" meditation, this involves mentally sending kindness and warm thoughts toward others by silently repeating a series of mantras like "may you be happy."
Best for anyone struggling with relationships.

→ WALKING MEDITATION
This type of meditation is exactly as it sounds—practicing mindfulness as you walk. But the focus is really on the steps itself, like the lifting and placement of each foot, as well as the shifting of body weight with each step.
Best for type-A personalities who have a hard time staying still.

LEARNING TO STAY PRESENT

Every year, I look back on the previous 12 months and think, wow, that went fast! And I begin the New Year resolving to start meditating, doing yoga, journaling and living in the moment, not frittering away my time on silly social media sites or dumb TV shows. Unfortunately, these goals tend to get lost in the frenzy of everyday life. That's why we designed this 2022 planner to help you (and me!) stay on track with a format that introduces a new practice every week. There are easy meditation exercises, simple yoga poses, and journaling, coloring and artistic prompts. By using this planner, you're assembling a "Mindfulness Toolbox" that will give you a variety of calming ways to start or end your day or to be your go-tos when things gets hectic. They'll help you enjoy life more, and make you less susceptible to anxiety and depression, improve your heart health and boost your immune system. So here's to making 2022 the best year ever.

Anne Marie O'Connor

"AND NOW WE WELCOME
THE NEW YEAR, FULL OF THINGS
THAT HAVE NEVER BEEN."

RAINER MARIA RILKE

2022
PLANNER

Record your activities and thoughts for every day of the week.

S

M

T

W

T

F

S

🌷 TO-DO LIST

_____

_____

_____

_____

Mood Chart

	S	M	T	W	T	F	S
☀							
🌤							
☁							
🌦							
🌧							
⛈							

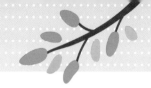

MINDFULNESS TOOLBOX BREATHING EXERCISE

At the beginning of the most stressful time of year, this simple breathing practice by Mallika Chopra, founder of the wellness website mallikachopra.com and author of *Just Breathe: Meditation, Mindfulness, Movement, and More*, is a good one to have in your toolbox. It can be used anywhere, anytime you feel overwhelmed.

→ **Close your eyes and take a deep breath in through your nose, feeling your lungs fill up.**

→ **Hold for a second, then breathe out, blowing out slowly from your mouth.**

→ **On your next breath, breathe in for three seconds, pause for two seconds, then breathe out for four seconds.**

→ **Continue with this pattern, or you can find a longer or shorter one that works for you.**

When did you use this exercise this week?

How did you feel afterward?

> "IF YOU WANT TO CONQUER THE ANXIETY OF LIFE, LIVE IN THE MOMENT, LIVE IN THE BREATH."
> **AMIT RAY**

Record your activities and thoughts for every day of the week.

S

M

T

W

T

F

S

🌷 **TO-DO LIST**

_____

_____

_____

_____

_____

Mood Chart

	S	M	T	W	T	F	S
☀							
⛅							
☁							
🌦							
🌧							
⛈							

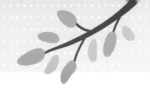

MINDFULNESS TOOLBOX JOURNALING EXERCISE

You probably have a list of presents to buy, cards to send and menus to plan.
On this page, make another list: of relationships you want to celebrate, moments
you hope to cherish, holiday treats you want to savor and other emotional presents you
hope to give during the season.

> "CHRISTMAS IS
> A SEASON FOR
> KINDLING THE FIRE
> FOR HOSPITALITY IN
> THE HALL, THE GENIAL
> FLAME OF CHARITY
> IN THE HEART."
> **WASHINGTON IRVING**

Record your activities and thoughts for every day of the week.

S

M

T FIRST DAY OF WINTER

W

T

F

S CHRISTMAS DAY

🌷 TO-DO LIST

	S	M	T	W	T	F	S
☀							
⛅							
☁							
🌦							
🌧							
⛈							

Mood Chart

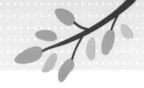

MINDFULNESS TOOLBOX COLORING EXERCISE

To make coloring mindful, follow these guidelines:

→ Set aside 15 minutes when you won't be interrupted.

→ Don't try to focus on anything specific; just pay attention to the colors, the patterns and the beauty you are creating.

→ Be aware of your thoughts without reacting to them. As you color these ornaments, be grateful for all the things that "decorate" your life and make it special.

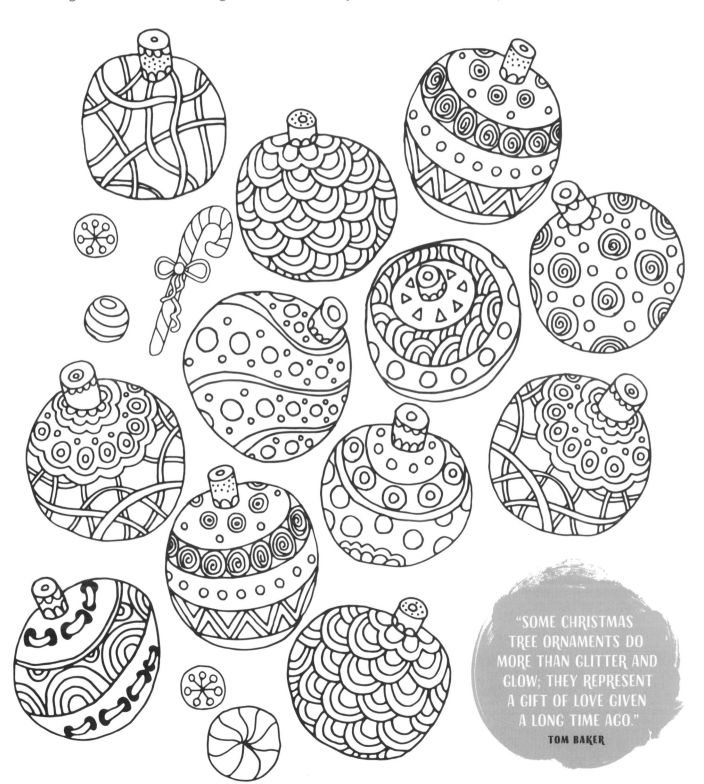

"SOME CHRISTMAS TREE ORNAMENTS DO MORE THAN GLITTER AND GLOW; THEY REPRESENT A GIFT OF LOVE GIVEN A LONG TIME AGO."

TOM BAKER

Record your activities and thoughts for every day of the week.

S

M

T

W

T

F

S   NEW YEAR'S DAY

TO-DO LIST

_____

_____

_____

_____

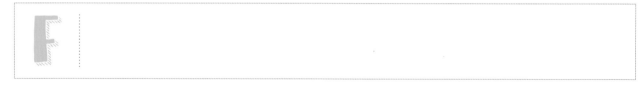

Mood Chart	S	M	T	W	T	F	S
☀							
⛅							
☁							
🌦							
🌧							
⛈							

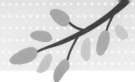

MINDFULNESS TOOLBOX JOURNALING EXERCISE

Pretend that you can give one (nonmaterial) gift to every child in the world.
What would you give them?

Why is that gift so important?

What has it meant in your life?

"WE CANNOT LIVE
ONLY FOR OURSELVES.
A THOUSAND FIBERS
CONNECT US WITH OUR
FELLOW MEN."
HERMAN MELVILLE

Record your activities and thoughts for every day of the week.

S

M

T

W

T

F

S

TO-DO LIST

_____

_____

_____

_____

_____

Mood Chart

	S	M	T	W	T	F	S
☀							
⛅							
☁							
🌧							
🌧							
⛈							

MINDFULNESS TOOLBOX ART EXERCISE

In the space below, create a vision board (either cut out or print out words and pictures) of things you're looking forward to in the year ahead.

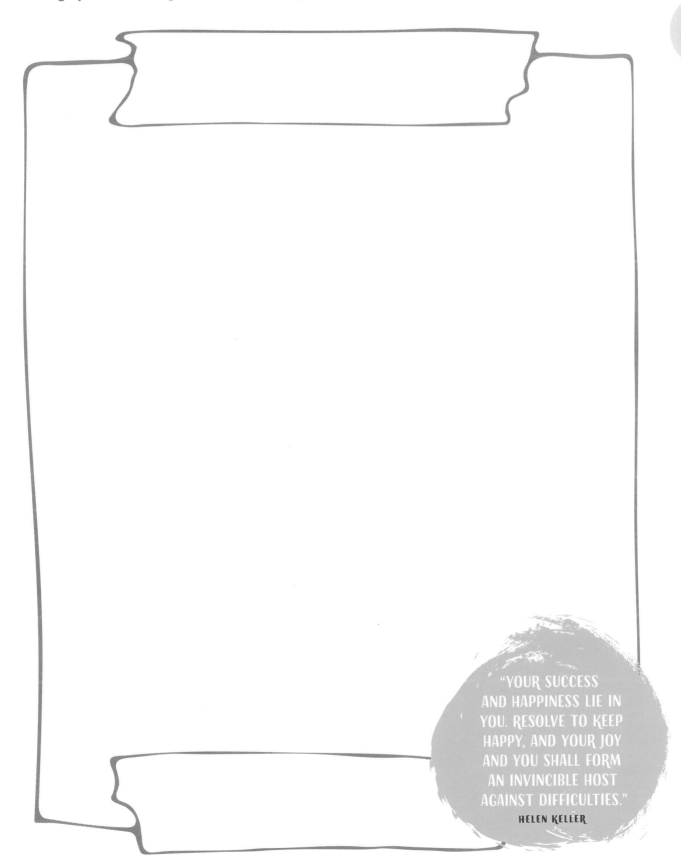

"YOUR SUCCESS AND HAPPINESS LIE IN YOU. RESOLVE TO KEEP HAPPY, AND YOUR JOY AND YOU SHALL FORM AN INVINCIBLE HOST AGAINST DIFFICULTIES."
HELEN KELLER

Record your activities and thoughts for every day of the week.

S

M

T

W

T

F

S

TO-DO LIST

_____

_____

_____

_____

_____

Mood Chart

	S	M	T	W	T	F	S
☀							
⛅							
☁							
🌧							
⛈							
🌥							

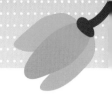

MINDFULNESS TOOLBOX JOURNALING EXERCISE
January is National Mentoring Month.
Journal about who in your life has been an important guide to you.

_____

_____

_____

_____

_____

_____

_____

_____

How did they inspire you?

_____

_____

_____

_____

_____

To whom have you passed on their lessons?

_____

_____

_____

_____

_____

_____

_____

"A MENTOR IS
SOMEONE WHO
ALLOWS YOU
TO SEE THE HOPE
INSIDE YOURSELF."
OPRAH WINFREY

Record your activities and thoughts for every day of the week.

S

M   MARTIN LUTHER KING JR. DAY

T

W

T

F

S

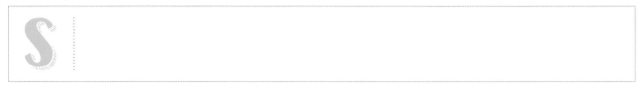 TO-DO LIST

_____

_____

_____

_____

_____

Mood Chart						
	S	M	T	W	T	F	S
☀							
⛅							
☁							
🌧							
🌧							
⛈							

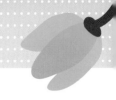

MINDFULNESS TOOLBOX JOURNALING EXERCISE

In celebration of Martin Luther King Jr.'s legacy, which we honor this week, reflect on his words below, and then journal about a grudge you haven't been able to let go of. What were the circumstances?

_____

_____

_____

_____

_____

_____

_____

_____

_____

_____

_____

How would you feel if you let go of it? Would your heart and spirit feel lighter?

_____

_____

_____

_____

_____

_____

_____

_____

_____

"I HAVE DECIDED TO STICK WITH LOVE. HATE IS TOO GREAT A BURDEN TO BEAR."
MARTIN LUTHER KING JR.

Record your activities and thoughts for every day of the week.

S

M

T

W

T

F

S

TO-DO LIST

_____

_____

_____

_____

_____

Mood Chart

	S	M	T	W	T	F	S
☀							
⛅							
☁							
🌧							
🌧							
⛈							

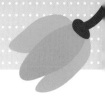

MINDFULNESS TOOLBOX JOURNALING EXERCISE

Set a mindful intention every morning this week before you get out of bed. (Some inspirations: What emotions would you like to nurture in your life? What would you like to let go of? What makes you your happiest self?) By starting the day with this thought, it's kept in the forefront of your conscious mind, making it much more likely it will happen.

How did setting an intention change your day?

Is this a helpful practice for you?

"OUR INTENTION
CREATES
OUR REALITY."
WAYNE DYER

Record your activities and thoughts for every day of the week.

S

M

T

W

T

F

S

TO-DO LIST

_____

_____

_____

_____

_____

Mood Chart							
	S	M	T	W	T	F	S
☀							
⛅							
☁							
🌧							
🌧							
⛈							

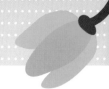

MINDFULNESS TOOLBOX JOURNALING EXERCISE

We tend to hibernate in winter.

How can you make this a more meaningful time?

What things that you find draining can you let go of?

What can you do to help yourself recharge?

"WHAT GOOD IS
THE WARMTH OF
SUMMER, WITHOUT
THE COLD OF
WINTER TO GIVE IT
SWEETNESS."
NATHANIEL BRANDEN

Record your activities and thoughts for every day of the week.

S

M

T

W

T

F

S

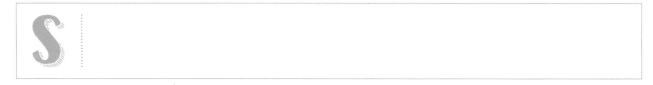

TO-DO LIST

_____

_____

_____

_____

Mood Chart

	S	M	T	W	T	F	S
☀							
⛅							
☁							
🌦							
🌧							
⛈							

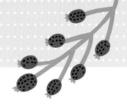

When we think positive thoughts about ourselves, we can overcome negative thinking and self-sabotaging behaviors. Write seven positive statements about yourself.

Repeat these affirmations to yourself—out loud—every morning this week.

1 _____

2 _____

3 _____

4 _____

5 _____

6 _____

7 _____

Has repeating affirmations uplifted your spirit or improved your self-image? How?

_____

_____

_____

_____

_____

"ONCE YOU REPLACE NEGATIVE THOUGHTS WITH POSITIVE ONES, YOU'LL START HAVING POSITIVE RESULTS."
WILLIE NELSON

Record your activities and thoughts for every day of the week.

S

M   VALENTINE'S DAY

T

W

T

F

S

TO-DO LIST

_____
_____
_____
_____
_____

Mood Chart

	S	M	T	W	T	F	S
☀							
⛅							
☁							
🌧							
🌧							
⛈							

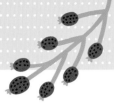

Write a love letter to yourself.

"LOVE RECOGNIZES NO BARRIERS. IT JUMPS HURDLES, LEAPS FENCES, PENETRATES WALLS TO ARRIVE AT ITS DESTINATION FULL OF HOPE."
MAYA ANGELOU

FEBRUARY 20 – FEBRUARY 26

Record your activities and thoughts for every day of the week.

S

M   PRESIDENTS' DAY

T

W

T

F

S

🪷 TO-DO LIST

_____

_____

_____

_____

_____

Mood Chart

	S	M	T	W	T	F	S
☀️							
⛅							
☁️							
🌦️							
🌧️							
⛈️							

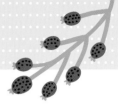

MINDFULNESS TOOLBOX COLORING EXERCISE

To make coloring mindful, follow these guidelines:

➔ Set aside 15 minutes when you won't be interrupted.

➔ Don't try to focus on anything specific; just pay attention to the colors, patterns and the beauty you are creating.

➔ Be aware of your thoughts without reacting to them. As you color these snowflakes, think about what makes you unique.

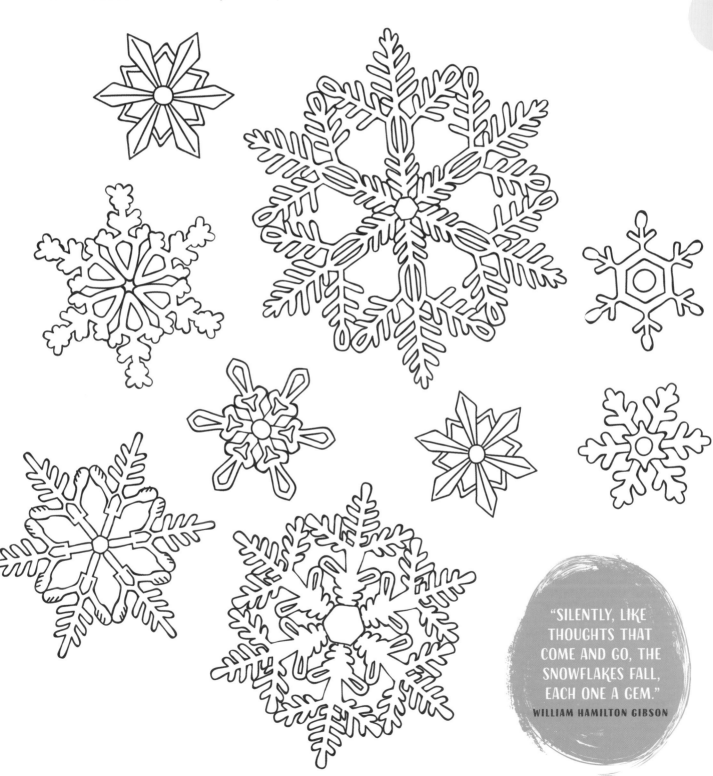

"SILENTLY, LIKE THOUGHTS THAT COME AND GO, THE SNOWFLAKES FALL, EACH ONE A GEM."
WILLIAM HAMILTON GIBSON

Record your activities and thoughts for every day of the week.

S

M

T

W READ ACROSS AMERICA DAY

T

F

S

TO-DO LIST

_____

_____

_____

_____

Mood Chart

	S	M	T	W	T	F	S
☀							
⛅							
☁							
🌧							
🌧							
⛈							

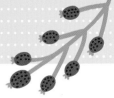

MINDFULNESS TOOLBOX RELAXATION EXERCISE

In honor of Read Across America Day, journal about your favorite character in a novel. What do you admire about him or her?

_____

_____

_____

_____

_____

_____

_____

What qualities helped him or her overcome obstacles?

_____

_____

_____

_____

_____

How has he or she inspired you in real life?

_____

_____

_____

_____

_____

"A READER LIVES
A THOUSAND LIVES
BEFORE HE DIES....
THE MAN WHO
NEVER READS LIVES
ONLY ONE."
GEORGE R.R. MARTIN

Record your activities and thoughts for every day of the week.

S

M

T

W

T

F

S

🍁 TO-DO LIST

_____

_____

_____

_____

Mood Chart

	S	M	T	W	T	F	S
☀							
⛅							
☁							
🌦							
🌧							
⛈							

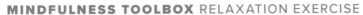

MINDFULNESS TOOLBOX RELAXATION EXERCISE

Do a progressive muscle relaxation for five minutes every day this week. Kathmandu, Nepal–based yoga teacher George Hughes explains how.

→ **Either sitting, lying down, or standing, take a moment to notice your body.**

→ **Tighten the muscles in your feet for a few seconds, then relax.**

→ **Tighten the muscles in your calves for a few seconds, then relax.**

→ **Now move on to your thighs, buttocks, abdomen, chest, arms and hands, tightening the muscles in them for a few moments, then relaxing.**

→ **Tighten and relax your neck and face.**

→ **Tighten your whole body for a few seconds, then let it go.**

Spend five minutes every day this week repeating this exercise. Also, try it in your daily life whenever you remember, especially when you feel stressed.

Did this exercise work for you? How did you feel afterward?

In what situations would it be helpful to practice it?

> "YOU NEED TO EMPTY YOUR MIND, AND RELAX EACH MUSCLE GROUP UNTIL YOU FEEL LIKE YOU ARE GOING TO MELT INTO THE FLOOR. THEN YOU JUST LET IT ALL GO. ALL THE EXPECTATIONS, ALL THE UNNEEDED WORRY."
> KASIE WEST

Record your activities and thoughts for every day of the week.

S DAYLIGHT SAVING TIME BEGINS

M

T

W

T

F

S

🌸 **TO-DO LIST**

_____

_____

_____

_____

_____

Mood Chart

	S	M	T	W	T	F	S
☀️							
⛅							
☁️							
🌧️							
🌧️							
⛈️							

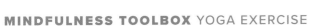

MINDFULNESS TOOLBOX YOGA EXERCISE

Always wanted to try yoga? Give this classic mindfulness activity a try with this simple cross-legged pose (sukhasana) for five minutes every day this week. A staple of meditators and yogis, "cross-legged pose can help you cultivate an inner stillness that carries over into your daily life," says A.J. Hanley, a Southold, New York–based yoga instructor. Here, she explains how to do it.

> **Sit tall on a blanket, your feet stacked under opposite knees. Close your eyes, soften your jaw and bring your attention to your breath and the sensations around it. Focus on your breath, but if thoughts come up, acknowledge them without irritation or judgment and then return to focusing on the breath.**

Did your mind wander while in cross-legged pose? What came up for you?

Did you notice a shift from your active or distracted mind toward a focused and centered mind?

How might this exercise be helpful to you in your daily life? Setting the tone for the day? Destressing after a day at work?

> "IN AN AGE OF CONSTANT MOVEMENT, NOTHING IS MORE URGENT THAN SITTING STILL."
> PICO IYER

Record your activities and thoughts for every day of the week.

S	FIRST DAY OF SPRING

M	

T	

W	

T	

F	

S	

❋ TO-DO LIST

_____

_____

_____

_____

Mood Chart	S	M	T	W	T	F	S
☀							
⛅							
☁							
🌧							
⛈							
⛆							

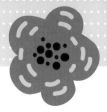

MINDFULNESS TOOLBOX COLORING EXERCISE

To make coloring mindful, follow these guidelines:

→ Set aside 15 minutes when you won't be interrupted.

→ Don't try to focus on anything specific; just pay attention to the colors, the patterns and the beauty you are creating.

→ Be aware of your thoughts without reacting to them. A mandala is a geometric figure that represents the universe; as you color it, contemplate the many forms of life that are reawakening now that it's spring.

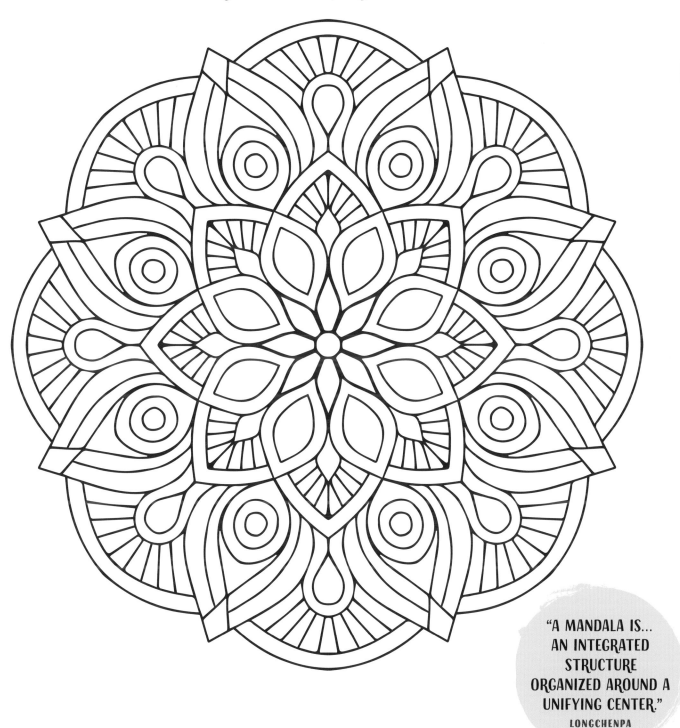

"A MANDALA IS...
AN INTEGRATED
STRUCTURE
ORGANIZED AROUND A
UNIFYING CENTER."
LONGCHENPA

Record your activities and thoughts for every day of the week.

S

M

T

W

T

F

S

🌸 TO-DO LIST

_____

_____

_____

_____

_____

Mood Chart							
	S	M	T	W	T	F	S
☀							
⛅							
☁							
🌧							
🌧							
⛈							

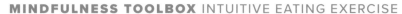

MINDFULNESS TOOLBOX INTUITIVE EATING EXERCISE

This week, practice mindful eating during one meal a day. That means focusing on what you're eating—no phone, no computer, no TV, no shoveling food in your mouth while standing at the kitchen counter or in the car.

> **Turn off your devices and sit with your food, truly tasting it, one bite at a time. Look at each forkful (or spoonful) before you eat it. Smell it. Then put it in your mouth, and pay attention to how each bite tastes, slowly chewing it and savoring its flavor.**

How did this change mealtimes for you?

_____

_____

_____

_____

_____

_____

_____

Did you find you ate less but enjoyed your food more?

_____

_____

_____

_____

_____

_____

"CONSCIOUS EATING IS A BIG STEP TOWARD CONSCIOUS LIVING."
NATASA PANTOVIC NUIT

Record your activities and thoughts for every day of the week.

S

M

T

W

T

F

S

🌷 TO-DO LIST

_____

_____

_____

_____

Mood Chart

	S	M	T	W	T	F	S
☀️							
🌤️							
☁️							
🌧️							
🌧️							
⛈️							

MINDFULNESS TOOLBOX JOURNALING EXERCISE

Write down five things you complain about the most.

1
2
3
4
5

Why do they bother you so much?

For each one, examine it from another perspective (for example, if your
kids dump all their stuff at the door, is it because they're excited to be home?
If your boss is always micromanaging you, consider the possibility that he
or she is feeling pressure from his or her boss).

1
2
3
4
5

Replace it with a thought about something you're grateful for.
Write it down here.

1
2
3
4
5

"WHEN YOU
ARISE IN THE MORNING,
THINK OF WHAT A
PRECIOUS PRIVILEGE IT
IS TO BE ALIVE—TO
BREATHE, TO THINK,
TO ENJOY, TO LOVE."
MARCUS AURELIUS

Record your activities and thoughts for every day of the week.

S

M

T

W

T

F

S | PASSOVER [FIRST DAY]

🌷 TO-DO LIST

_____

_____

_____

_____

_____

Mood Chart

	S	M	T	W	T	F	S
☀							
⛅							
☁							
🌦							
🌧							
⛈							

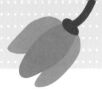

April showers bring May flowers, so it's a perfect time to try a smell-the-flowers practice:

> **Take five minutes to focus on and relish the smell of something—a flower, a plant, the grass, your backyard. Repeat several times during the week.**

Describe the scent.

_____

_____

_____

_____

_____

What memories does it evoke?

_____

_____

_____

_____

_____

What other ways can you find to savor nature in your everyday life?

_____

_____

_____

_____

"A SINGLE GENTLE RAIN MAKES THE GRASS MANY SHADES GREENER."
HENRY DAVID THOREAU

Record your activities and thoughts for every day of the week.

S | EASTER

M |

T |

W |

T |

F | EARTH DAY

S |

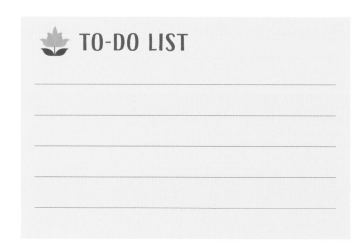

🌷 TO-DO LIST

_____

_____

_____

_____

Mood Chart	S	M	T	W	T	F	S
☀							
⛅							
☁							
🌧							
⛆							
⛈							

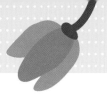

MINDFULNESS TOOLBOX COLORING EXERCISE

To make coloring mindful, follow these guidelines:

→ Set aside 15 minutes when you won't be interrupted.

→ Don't try to focus on anything specific; just pay attention to the colors, the patterns and the beauty you are creating.

→ Be aware of your thoughts without reacting to them. Eggs symbolize birth and renewal; as you color, think about what new things you want to bring into your life.

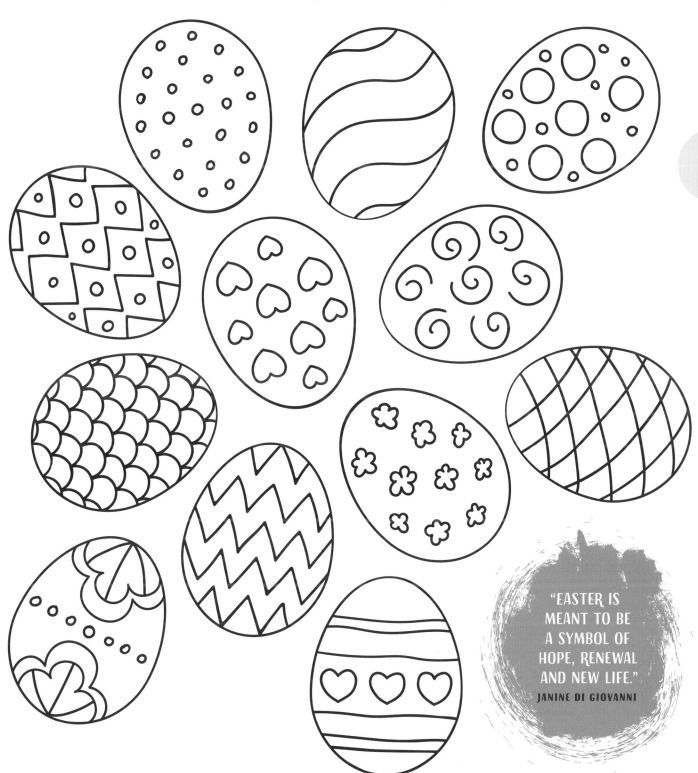

"EASTER IS MEANT TO BE A SYMBOL OF HOPE, RENEWAL AND NEW LIFE."
JANINE DI GIOVANNI

Record your activities and thoughts for every day of the week.

S

M

T

W

T

F

S

🌸 TO-DO LIST

_____

_____

_____

_____

_____

Mood Chart

	S	M	T	W	T	F	S
☀️							
🌤️							
☁️							
🌧️							
⛈️							
🌩️							

MINDFULNESS TOOLBOX JOURNALING EXERCISE

What are some ways you can be kinder?

How will it change how you feel?

What's preventing you from doing it?

"A SINGLE ACT OF
KINDNESS THROWS
OUT ROOTS IN ALL
DIRECTIONS, AND THE
ROOTS SPRING UP AND
MAKE NEW TREES."
AMELIA EARHART

Record your activities and thoughts for every day of the week.

S — MAY DAY

M

T

W

T

F

S

🌷 TO-DO LIST

_____

_____

_____

_____

_____

Mood Chart

	S	M	T	W	T	F	S
☀							
⛅							
☁							
🌧							
🌧							
⛈							

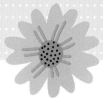

MINDFULNESS TOOLBOX JOURNALING EXERCISE

May Day is a time for celebrating the joys of spring. Describe your favorite place to be outside. Where is it? What does it look like? What does it smell like?

_____

_____

_____

_____

_____

_____

_____

_____

_____

_____

_____

_____

How do you feel when you're there?

_____

_____

_____

_____

_____

_____

_____

_____

_____

"THE BEAUTIFUL SPRING CAME, AND WHEN NATURE RESUMES HER LOVELINESS, THE HUMAN SOUL IS APT TO REVIVE ALSO."

HARRIET ANN JACOBS

Record your activities and thoughts for every day of the week.

S MOTHER'S DAY

M

T

W

T

F

S

🪷 TO-DO LIST

_____

_____

_____

_____

_____

Mood Chart

	S	M	T	W	T	F	S
☀							
⛅							
☁							
🌧							
🌧							
⛈							

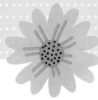

MINDFULNESS TOOLBOX MEDITATION EXERCISE

In honor of Mother's Day, reflect on what you love most about your mom.

What have you always wanted to tell her?

What are some of the similarities between you and her that you most cherish?

What similarities do you dislike?

"MOTHERHOOD:
ALL LOVE
BEGINS AND
ENDS THERE."
ROBERT BROWNING

Record your activities and thoughts for every day of the week.

S

M

T

W

T

F

S

🪷 TO-DO LIST

_____

_____

_____

_____

_____

Mood Chart

	S	M	T	W	T	F	S
☀️							
⛅							
☁️							
🌧️							
⛈️							
🌩️							

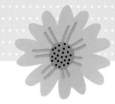

MINDFULNESS TOOLBOX MEDITATION EXERCISE

To enhance your awareness in your daily life, meditation and yoga teacher George Hughes suggests trying a sound meditation. Here's how.

→ **In a comfortable position, seated or lying down, take a few deep breaths.**

→ **Bring your attention to any sounds you hear. You do not need to strain your ears or hang onto them; simply notice whatever sounds come to you.**

→ **After a short while, relax once again and focus on your breath.**

→ **Alternate between noticing sounds and noticing breath for five minutes.**

→ **Spend five minutes every day this week repeating this exercise.**

What sounds did you hear?

_____

_____

How did they make you feel?

_____

_____

_____

What sounds do you find particularly soothing?

_____

_____

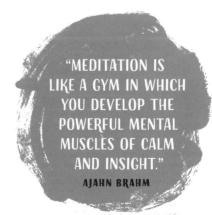

"MEDITATION IS LIKE A GYM IN WHICH YOU DEVELOP THE POWERFUL MENTAL MUSCLES OF CALM AND INSIGHT."
AJAHN BRAHM

Record your activities and thoughts for every day of the week.

S

M

T

W

T

F

S

TO-DO LIST

_____

_____

_____

_____

_____

Mood Chart

	S	M	T	W	T	F	S
☼							
⛅							
☁							
🌦							
🌧							
⛈							

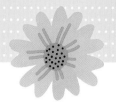

MINDFULNESS TOOLBOX COLORING EXERCISE

To make coloring mindful, follow these guidelines:

→ Set aside 15 minutes when you won't be interrupted.

→ Don't try to focus on anything specific; just pay attention to the colors, the patterns and the beauty you are creating.

→ Be aware of your thoughts without reacting to them. While you color in these flowers, contemplate openings: of petals, thoughts and minds.

"MINDS ARE LIKE FLOWERS; THEY OPEN ONLY WHEN THE TIME IS RIGHT."
STEPHEN RICHARDS

Record your activities and thoughts for every day of the week.

S

M   MEMORIAL DAY

T

W

T

F

S

TO-DO LIST

_____

_____

_____

_____

_____

Mood Chart

	S	M	T	W	T	F	S
☀							
⛅							
☁							
🌧							
🌧							
⛈							

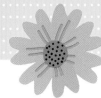

MINDFULNESS TOOLBOX JOURNALING EXERCISE

Recall a painful event from your childhood. Describe it in detail.

How has it affected your life?

How would you comfort your younger self?

"EXPERIENCING TERRIBLE PAIN OPENS OUR HEARTS AND MINDS TO EXPRESS COMPASSION FOR OTHER PEOPLE AND COMMUNION WITH OURSELVES."

KILROY J. OLDSTER

Record your activities and thoughts for every day of the week.

S

M

T

W

T

F

S

🌷 TO-DO LIST

_____

_____

_____

_____

Mood Chart						
	S	M	T	W	T	F	S
☀							
⛅							
☁							
🌧							
🌧							
⛈							

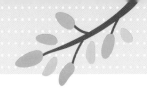

MINDFULNESS TOOLBOX JOURNALING EXERCISE

Try the Raisin Exercise, which was developed by Jon Kabat-Zinn, PhD, the founder of mindfulness-based stress reduction (MBSR), as a first meditation for his clients. It will help you engage the five senses, to learn the basics of mindfulness, reduce stress, become more attentive and savor small pleasures.

1 **Take a raisin (or any food) in your hand. Look at it as if you've never seen it before. Observe its shape, its creases, its colors.**

2 **After a minute or so, roll the raisin between your fingers. Feel how soft it is; take note of its texture.**

3 **Then smell the raisin. Contemplate its sweetness, its fruitiness.**

4 **Next, bring the raisin close to your ear. Rub it, squeeze it, listen for any sound it makes.**

5 **Put the raisin in your mouth and explore it with your tongue. Feel the texture, the shape and the sensations it creates. Then bite down on it, and notice its taste. Finally, swallow it, noting the path it takes down your throat and the aftertaste it leaves.**

Spend five minutes every day this week repeating this exercise. Also, try it at regular meals, noticing and appreciating the foods on your plate.

"THE FIRST STEP TOWARD CHANGE IS AWARENESS."
NATHANIEL BRANDEN

Record your activities and thoughts for every day of the week.

S

M

T

W

T

F

S

🪷 **TO-DO LIST**

Mood Chart							
	S	M	T	W	T	F	S
☀️							
🌤️							
☁️							
🌧️							
🌧️							
⛈️							

MINDFULNESS TOOLBOX COLORING EXERCISE

To make coloring mindful, follow these guidelines:

→ Set aside 15 minutes when you won't be interrupted.

→ Don't try to focus on anything specific; just pay attention to the colors, the patterns and the beauty you are creating.

→ Be aware of your thoughts without reacting to them. While you color the butterflies, think of how their wings allow them to float above the world, and allow your thoughts to do the same, without becoming entangled by anything in their path.

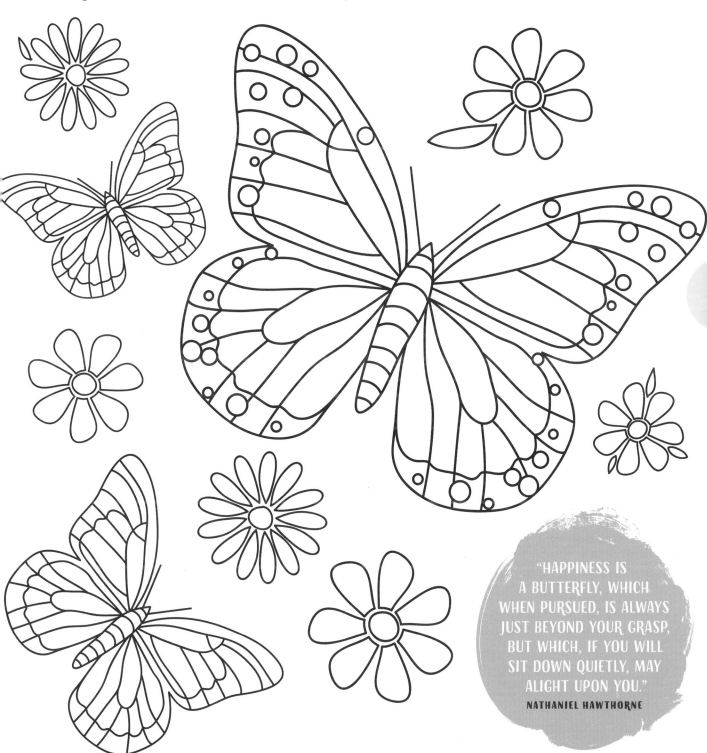

"HAPPINESS IS A BUTTERFLY, WHICH WHEN PURSUED, IS ALWAYS JUST BEYOND YOUR GRASP, BUT WHICH, IF YOU WILL SIT DOWN QUIETLY, MAY ALIGHT UPON YOU."

NATHANIEL HAWTHORNE

Record your activities and thoughts for every day of the week.

S   FATHER'S DAY
JUNETEENTH

M

T   FIRST DAY OF SUMMER

W

T

F

S

 TO-DO LIST

_____

_____

_____

_____

Mood Chart

	S	M	T	W	T	F	S
☀							
⛅							
☁							
🌧							
🌧							
⛈							

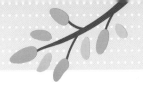

MINDFULNESS TOOLBOX JOURNALING EXERCISE
In honor of Father's Day, write a thank-you note to your dad or other father figure.

What five things are you most grateful to him for?

1

2

3

4

5

"DADS ARE MOST
ORDINARY MEN
TURNED BY LOVE INTO
HEROES, ADVENTURERS,
STORY-TELLERS, AND
SINGERS OF SONG."
PAM BROWN

Record your activities and thoughts for every day of the week.

S

M

T

W

T

F

S

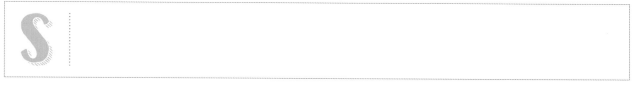 TO-DO LIST

_____

_____

_____

_____

Mood Chart	S	M	T	W	T	F	S
☀							
⛅							
☁							
🌧							
⛈							
🌩							

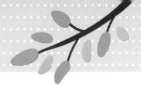

MINDFULNESS TOOLBOX JOURNALING EXERCISE

Every morning this week, write down any dream (even if just a part of a dream) as soon as you wake up. What do you think it means?

"DREAMS ARE
ILLUSTRATIONS...
FROM THE BOOK
YOUR SOUL IS
WRITING ABOUT YOU."
MARSHA NORMAN

Record your activities and thoughts for every day of the week.

S

M INDEPENDENCE DAY

T

W

T

F

S

 TO-DO LIST

	S	M	T	W	T	F	S
Mood Chart							
☀							
⛅							
☁							
🌧							
⛈							
🌩							

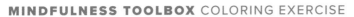

MINDFULNESS TOOLBOX COLORING EXERCISE

To make coloring mindful, follow these guidelines:

→ Set aside 15 minutes when you won't be interrupted.

→ Don't try to focus on anything specific; just pay attention to the colors, the patterns and the beauty you are creating.

→ Be aware of your thoughts without reacting to them. While you color in the fireworks, think about the freedom and beauty you enjoy in your life.

"HUMANITY HAS WON ITS BATTLE. LIBERTY NOW HAS A COUNTRY."
MARQUIS DE LAFAYETTE

Record your activities and thoughts for every day of the week.

S

M

T

W

T

F

S

🌸 TO-DO LIST

_____

_____

_____

_____

Mood Chart							
	S	M	T	W	T	F	S
☀							
⛅							
☁							
🌦							
🌧							
⛈							

Meditating using a mantra can be helpful for people who have trouble focusing on their breath, or can be a way to mix up your usual practice. Alice Domar, PhD, executive director of the Domar Center for Mind/Body Health, explains how to get started.

→ **Sit in a comfortable chair, in a quiet spot.**

→ **Breathe like you normally would, in and out of your nose. Your eyes can be open or closed.**

→ **Pick a mantra. It can be as simple as "peace," "shalom" or "the Lord is my shepherd." It can be either religious or secular, as long as it relaxes you. Repeat it with each inhale, and with each exhale.**

→ **If your mind wanders, don't stress— simply return your focus to chanting the mantra and your breathing.**

→ **Initially, you may only be able to do this meditation for five minutes at a time, but eventually try building it up to 10, 20 or even 30 minutes.**

"I VISUALIZE WHAT I WANT THROUGH MEDITATION. THE PROCESS OF MEDITATING IS A GREAT WAY OF MAKING SURE I HAVE MY PRIORITIES SORTED."
SHILPA SHETTY

Record your activities and thoughts for every day of the week.

S

M

T

W

T

F

S

🪷 TO-DO LIST

_____

_____

_____

_____

_____

Mood Chart

	S	M	T	W	T	F	S
☀							
⛅							
☁							
🌦							
🌧							
⛈							

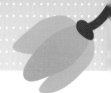

MINDFULNESS TOOLBOX JOURNALING EXERCISE

What's your favorite childhood memory of summer? What do you most look forward to every summer? What's on your must-do list for this summer?

"EVERYTHING GOOD, EVERYTHING MAGICAL HAPPENS BETWEEN THE MONTHS OF JUNE AND AUGUST."
JENNY HAN

Record your activities and thoughts for every day of the week.

S

M

T

W

T

F

S

TO-DO LIST

_____

_____

_____

_____

Mood Chart

	S	M	T	W	T	F	S
☀							
⛅							
☁							
🌦							
🌧							
⛈							

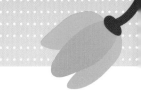

MINDFULNESS TOOLBOX MEDITATION EXERCISE

A walking meditation is an easy, accessible way to invite mindfulness into your daily life at any time, according to meditation and yoga teacher George Hughes. Try this for five minutes each day this week (you can also do it for longer).

→ **Find a place where you can be undisturbed while you walk. A park, a place in nature or your living room or office can be good practice spaces. There is no need to slow down your movements or exaggerate them—just walk in a relaxed, natural manner.**

→ **As you walk, notice what it feels like as your feet strike and lift from the ground. How do your legs feel as you move? Your arms? Is there a breeze? What do you see, hear, smell, taste or feel?**

→ **The point is to observe what we don't usually notice when we walk. Try not to judge, list or take notes, and simply "be" in the experience of walking.**

What did you see that you don't usually see?

"IN EVERY WALK WITH NATURE ONE RECEIVES FAR MORE THAN HE SEEKS."
JOHN MUIR

Record your activities and thoughts for every day of the week.

S

M

T

W

T

F

S

🪷 TO-DO LIST

Mood Chart

	S	M	T	W	T	F	S
☀️							
⛅							
☁️							
🌧️							
🌧️							
⛈️							

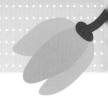

MINDFULNESS TOOLBOX COLORING EXERCISE

To make coloring mindful, follow these guidelines:

→ Set aside 15 minutes when you won't be interrupted.

→ Don't try to focus on anything specific; just pay attention to the colors, the patterns and the beauty you are creating.

→ Be aware of your thoughts without reacting to them. As you color this picture, think about how you feel in the water, weightless and free.

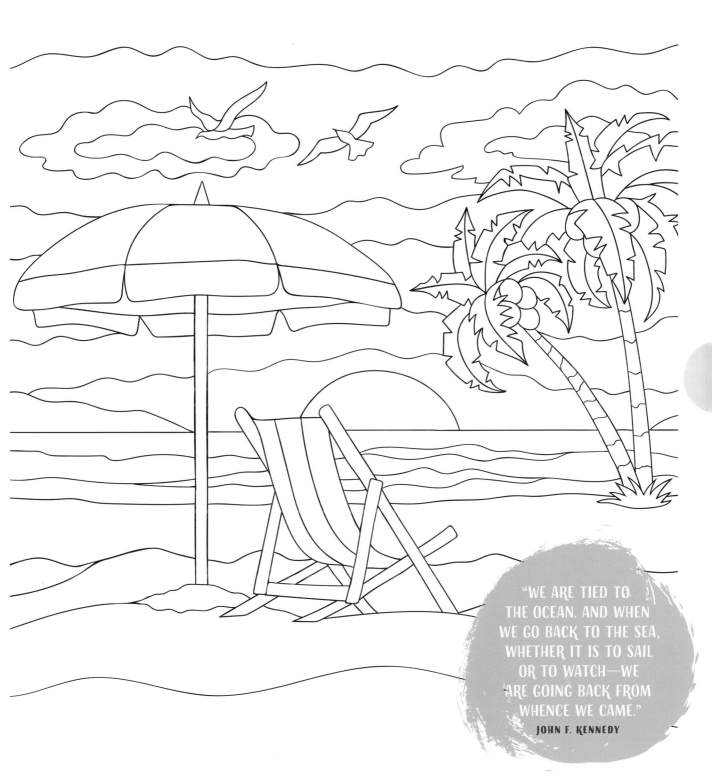

"WE ARE TIED TO THE OCEAN. AND WHEN WE GO BACK TO THE SEA, WHETHER IT IS TO SAIL OR TO WATCH—WE ARE GOING BACK FROM WHENCE WE CAME."

JOHN F. KENNEDY

Record your activities and thoughts for every day of the week.

S

M

T

W

T

F

S

TO-DO LIST

_____

_____

_____

_____

Mood Chart

	S	M	T	W	T	F	S
☀							
⛅							
☁							
🌦							
🌧							
⛈							

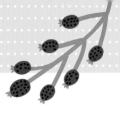

MINDFULNESS TOOLBOX JOURNALING EXERCISE

Who are the most important people in your support system?
What do you rely on each of them for?

How have they made your life better and more fulfilling?

What was a hard time they helped you get through?

"BE STRONG, BE
FEARLESS, BE BEAUTIFUL.
AND BELIEVE THAT
ANYTHING IS POSSIBLE
WHEN YOU HAVE THE
RIGHT PEOPLE THERE
TO SUPPORT YOU."
MISTY COPELAND

Record your activities and thoughts for every day of the week.

S

M

T

W

T

F

S

🌷 TO-DO LIST

_____

_____

_____

_____

_____

Mood Chart

	S	M	T	W	T	F	S
☀							
⛅							
☁							
🌧							
🌧							
⛈							

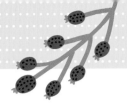

MINDFULNESS TOOLBOX YOGA EXERCISE

Do legs-up-the-wall pose (viparita karani) for 10 minutes every evening before bed this week. "Legs-up-the-wall pose can relax body and mind, helping you sleep more soundly," says A.J. Hanley, a yoga instructor in Southold, New York.

→ **Sit sideways against a wall.**

→ **Gently turn to swing your legs up onto the wall as you lie back, resting your head and shoulders on the floor.**

→ **Close your eyes and breathe slowly and deeply, scanning the body for any areas of tension for at least 10 minutes.**

Were there areas of your body that felt tight or uncomfortable?

List any reasons that you might be holding tension in those areas. Any stress about the day ahead? Offloading your to-do list before bed has been shown to make it easier to fall asleep.

"YOGA HAS A SLY, CLEVER WAY OF SHORT-CIRCUITING THE MENTAL PATTERNS THAT CAUSE ANXIETY."
BAXTER BELL

Record your activities and thoughts for every day of the week.

S

M

T

W

T

F

S

🌷 **TO-DO LIST**

_____

_____

_____

_____

Mood Chart							
	S	M	T	W	T	F	S
☀							
⛅							
☁							
🌦							
🌧							
⛈							

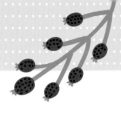

Make a list of all your major accomplishments.
Why are you proud of them?

What do they represent in your life?

What do they tell you about what you can make happen in the future?

"HAPPINESS LIES
IN THE JOY OF
ACHIEVEMENT AND
THE THRILL OF
CREATIVE EFFORT."
FRANKLIN D. ROOSEVELT

Record your activities and thoughts for every day of the week.

S

M

T

W

T

F

S

TO-DO LIST

_____

_____

_____

_____

_____

Mood Chart

	S	M	T	W	T	F	S
☀							
⛅							
☁							
🌧							
🌧							
⛈							

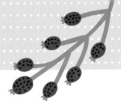

MINDFULNESS TOOLBOX COLORING EXERCISE

To make coloring mindful, follow these guidelines:

→ Set aside 15 minutes when you won't be interrupted.

→ Don't try to focus on anything specific; just pay attention to the colors, the patterns and the beauty you are creating.

→ Be aware of your thoughts without reacting to them. As you color these circles, think about their meaning, as symbols of both the infinite and the interconnectedness of all things.

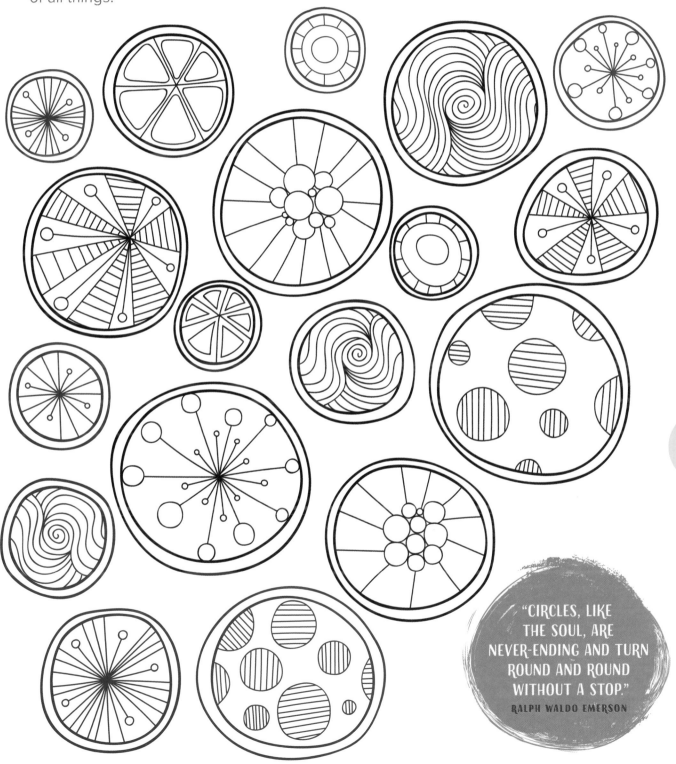

"CIRCLES, LIKE THE SOUL, ARE NEVER-ENDING AND TURN ROUND AND ROUND WITHOUT A STOP."
RALPH WALDO EMERSON

Record your activities and thoughts for every day of the week.

S

M   LABOR DAY

T

W

T

F

S

🍁 **TO-DO LIST**

_____

_____

_____

_____

_____

Mood Chart

	S	M	T	W	T	F	S
☀							
⛅							
☁							
🌦							
🌧							
⛈							

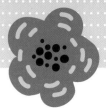

MINDFULNESS TOOLBOX JOURNALING EXERCISE

If you could take a year off work (but still get paid), what would you do?

Where would you go? Who would you spend it with?

What changes can you make in your real life so it would most resemble the fantasy?

> "TWENTY YEARS
> FROM NOW YOU WILL
> BE MORE DISAPPOINTED
> BY THE THINGS YOU
> DIDN'T DO THAN BY
> THE THINGS YOU DID."
> **MARK TWAIN**

Record your activities and thoughts for every day of the week.

S

M

T

W

T

F

S

❀ TO-DO LIST

Mood Chart							
	S	M	T	W	T	F	S
☀							
⛅							
☁							
🌦							
🌧							
⛈							

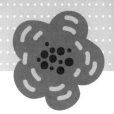

MINDFULNESS TOOLBOX JOURNALING EXERCISE

Even if it's been a long time since you completed a homework assignment
or wrote a book report, the end of summer still reminds us of going back to school.

What would you like to learn this year?

What books would you like to read?

What adult version of an extracurricular activity would you like to get involved with?

Record your activities and thoughts for every day of the week.

S

M

T

W   INTERNATIONAL DAY OF PEACE

T   FIRST DAY OF AUTUMN

F

S

🍁 TO-DO LIST

_____

_____

_____

_____

_____

Mood Chart

	S	M	T	W	T	F	S
☀							
⛅							
☁							
🌦							
🌧							
⛈							

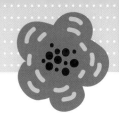

MINDFULNESS TOOLBOX JOURNALING EXERCISE

The U.N. General Assembly has designated September 21 as a day devoted to the ideals of peace among people and nations.

Reflect on the concept of peace and its relationship to mindfulness in your life.

What does world peace look like to you?

What can you do on an individual level to promote peace in your small corner of the universe?

How do you feel when you are living in peace instead of in anger and quarreling?

"PEACE BEGINS
WITH A SMILE."
MOTHER TERESA

Record your activities and thoughts for every day of the week.

S

M   FIRST DAY OF ROSH HASHANA

T

W

T

F

S

✿ TO-DO LIST

_____

_____

_____

_____

Mood Chart

	S	M	T	W	T	F	S
☀							
⛅							
☁							
🌧							
🌧							
⛈							

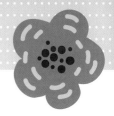

MINDFULNESS TOOLBOX BREATHING EXERCISE

This breathing exercise can be done anywhere, and can help bring stillness and awareness to even stressful situations, says George Hughes, a yoga and meditation teacher in Kathmandu, Nepal.

→ **Lie down on your back or sit comfortably in a chair (this can be done standing up). Place your hands near your waist, with thumbs at your lower ribs and pinkies at your hips.**

→ **Breathe slowly and deeply three times, focusing on your hands, allowing your lower belly to expand and contract.**

→ **Move your hands up and place them around the sides of your chest. Breathe slowly and deeply three times, allowing your chest to expand and contract.**

→ **Place your fingers at your collarbones. Breathe slowly and deeply three times into your upper chest, expanding and contracting the space under your hands and the space between your shoulder blades.**

→ **Now breathe normally, allowing yourself to notice whatever there is to notice. Repeat this exercise for five minutes every day this week.**

When did you do this exercise? Did you feel different afterward? How so? When do you think it might be helpful to do?

"BREATHING EASILY AND FULLY IS ONE OF THE BASIC PLEASURES OF BEING ALIVE."
ALEXANDER LOWEN

Record your activities and thoughts for every day of the week.

S

M

T

W   YOM KIPPUR

T

F

S

🪷 **TO-DO LIST**

_____

_____

_____

_____

_____

Mood Chart							
	S	M	T	W	T	F	S
☀️							
⛅							
☁️							
🌧️							
⛈️							
☔							

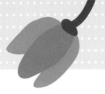

MINDFULNESS TOOLBOX COLORING EXERCISE

To make coloring mindful, follow these guidelines:

→ Set aside 15 minutes when you won't be interrupted.

→ Don't try to focus on anything specific; just pay attention to the colors, the patterns and the beauty you are creating.

→ Be aware of your thoughts without reacting to them. As you color these leaves, think about how you can show off your most vivid colors.

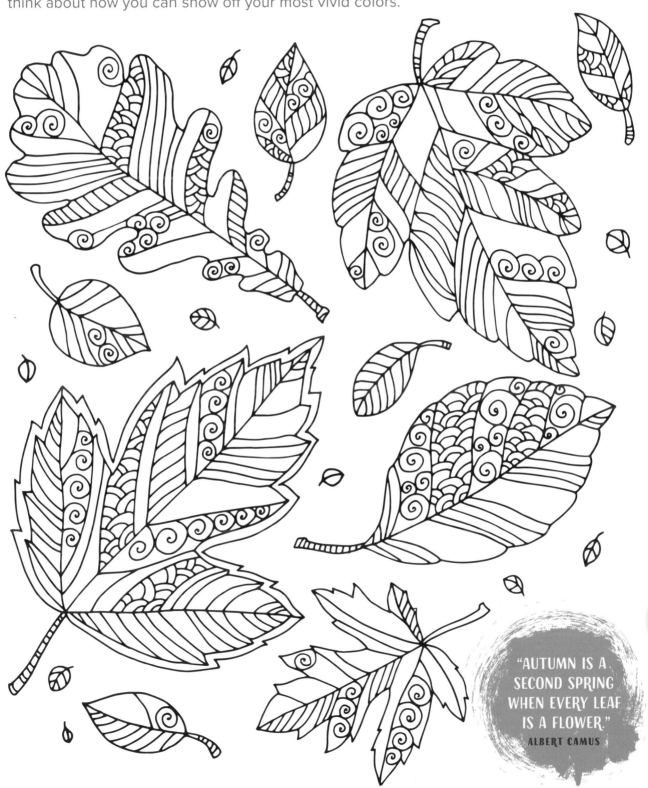

"AUTUMN IS A SECOND SPRING WHEN EVERY LEAF IS A FLOWER."
ALBERT CAMUS

OCTOBER 9 – OCTOBER 15

Record your activities and thoughts for every day of the week.

S

M   COLUMBUS DAY/INDIGENOUS PEOPLES' DAY

T

W

T

F

S

🍂 TO-DO LIST

	Mood Chart						
	S	M	T	W	T	F	S
☀							
⛅							
☁							
🌧							
🌧							
⛈							

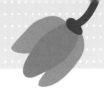

MINDFULNESS TOOLBOX JOURNALING EXERCISE

The Proust Questionnaire was popularized by French writer Marcel Proust, who believed these questions revealed one's true character. Here is our (abbreviated) version.

What is your idea of perfect happiness?

_____

_____

What is your most treasured possession?

_____

_____

What or who is the greatest love of your life?

_____

_____

When and where were you the happiest?

_____

_____

What is your greatest fear?

_____

_____

Which talent would you most like to have?

_____

_____

Where would you like to live?

_____

_____

On what occasions do you lie?

_____

_____

Which words or phrases do you most overuse?

_____

_____

What is your motto?

_____

_____

"WITHOUT
SELF-KNOWLEDGE...
MAN CANNOT
BE FREE."
G.I. GURDJIEFF

Record your activities and thoughts for every day of the week.

S

M

T

W

T

F

S

TO-DO LIST

_____

_____

_____

_____

_____

Mood Chart

	S	M	T	W	T	F	S
☀							
⛅							
☁							
🌦							
🌧							
⛈							

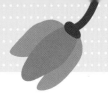

Chimes are often incorporated into meditation practices—the sound reminds you to stop for a moment and consciously breathe in and out three times. And of course, there's an app for that (more than one, in fact).

> **→ Download MindBell for Android or Mindfulness Bell for iOS to your phone and set the chime to sound at specific times or intervals (say, once an hour, or three times a day). Breathe in and out through your nose three times.**
>
>
>
> **→ This week, set a chime to ring at least three times a day.**

What were you doing when the chime rang?

How were you feeling beforehand?

How did you feel afterward?

"LISTENING TO THE BELL, I FEEL THE AFFLICTIONS IN ME BEGIN TO DISSOLVE. MY MIND BECOMES CALM, MY BODY RELAXED AND A SMILE IS BORN ON MY LIPS."
THÍCH NHẤT HẠNH

Record your activities and thoughts for every day of the week.

S

M

T

W

T

F

S

🌷 TO-DO LIST

_____

_____

_____

_____

Mood Chart							
	S	M	T	W	T	F	S
☀							
⛅							
☁							
🌧							
🌧							
⛈							

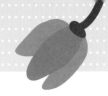

MINDFULNESS TOOLBOX JOURNALING EXERCISE

Every day this week, write about someone you're grateful is in your life. Why do you love him or her? What does he or she bring into your life? How has he or she influenced you?

Sunday

Monday

Tuesday

Wednesday

Thursday

Friday

Saturday

"MANY PEOPLE WILL WALK IN AND OUT OF YOUR LIFE, BUT ONLY TRUE FRIENDS WILL LEAVE FOOTPRINTS IN YOUR HEART."
ELEANOR ROOSEVELT

Record your activities and thoughts for every day of the week.

S

M HALLOWEEN

T

W

T

F

S

🪷 TO-DO LIST

Mood Chart							
	S	M	T	W	T	F	S
☀️							
⛅							
☁️							
🌧️							
🌧️							
⛈️							

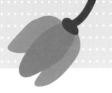

MINDFULNESS TOOLBOX COLORING EXERCISE

To make coloring mindful, follow these guidelines:

→ Set aside 15 minutes when you won't be interrupted.

→ Don't try to focus on anything specific; just pay attention to the colors, the patterns and the beauty you are creating.

→ Be aware of your thoughts without reacting to them. As you color this spiderweb, think about the role of patience and planning in our lives.

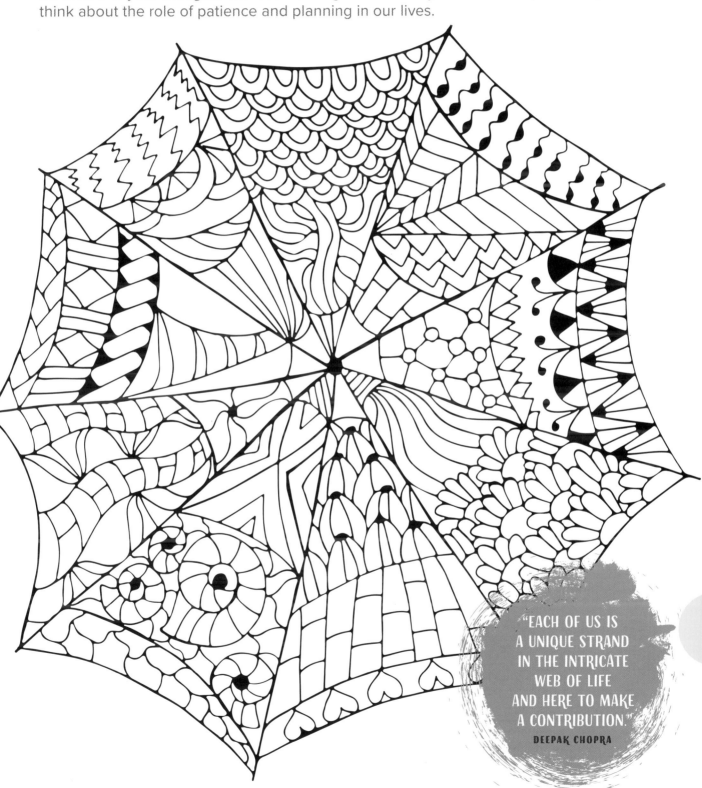

"EACH OF US IS A UNIQUE STRAND IN THE INTRICATE WEB OF LIFE AND HERE TO MAKE A CONTRIBUTION."

DEEPAK CHOPRA

Record your activities and thoughts for every day of the week.

S | DAYLIGHT SAVING TIME ENDS

M

T | ELECTION DAY

W

T

F | VETERANS DAY

S

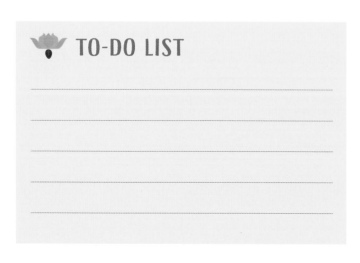
TO-DO LIST

_____

_____

_____

_____

Mood Chart

	S	M	T	W	T	F	S
☀							
⛅							
☁							
🌦							
🌧							
⛈							

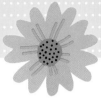

MINDFULNESS TOOLBOX JOURNALING EXERCISE

This week, when did you find it difficult to be "in the moment" and attentive to loved ones?

What was distracting you? What do you think you missed?

Why do you want to be present for them?

Are there things in your life you regret not being present for?

"MINDFULNESS IS SIMPLY BEING AWARE OF WHAT IS HAPPENING RIGHT NOW WITHOUT WISHING IT WERE DIFFERENT."
JAMES BARAZ

Record your activities and thoughts for every day of the week.

S

M

T

W

T

F

S

🌷 TO-DO LIST

_____

_____

_____

_____

Mood Chart	S	M	T	W	T	F	S
☀️							
⛅							
☁️							
🌦️							
🌧️							
⛈️							

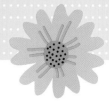

This week, take a self-compassion pause at least once a day, suggests George Hughes, a yoga and meditation teacher in Kathmandu, Nepal. "Just take a few minutes each day to recognize some of your own good qualities. This can seem selfish or self-centered in today's society, but the kinder and more compassionate we are to ourselves in our daily lives, the easier it is to be kind and compassionate to others." Here's how to show love to ourselves.

→ **While seated comfortably, take a few deep breaths.**

→ **Bring to mind five good things you have done in your life. These don't have to be big or even recent things, but try to think of different ones every time. They can be as simple as "I ate today, so I have the energy to get through the day," or "I remembered a loved one's birthday."**

→ **Sit with the first of these things for several breaths, then move onto the next.**

→ **Feel compassion and love, whether it is toward yourself or another. Remembering these expressions of your goodness can help us be a little easier on ourselves and allow us to blossom into the kind, compassionate, loving being within.**

What did you realize about yourself that you weren't aware of before doing this exercise?

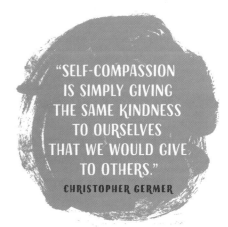

"SELF-COMPASSION IS SIMPLY GIVING THE SAME KINDNESS TO OURSELVES THAT WE WOULD GIVE TO OTHERS."
CHRISTOPHER GERMER

Record your activities and thoughts for every day of the week.

S

M

T

W

T   THANKSGIVING

F

S

🌷 TO-DO LIST

_____

_____

_____

_____

Mood Chart

	S	M	T	W	T	F	S
☀							
⛅							
☁							
🌦							
🌧							
⛈							

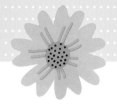

MINDFULNESS TOOLBOX COLORING EXERCISE

To make coloring mindful, follow these guidelines:

→ Set aside 15 minutes when you won't be interrupted.

→ Don't try to focus on anything specific; just pay attention to the colors, the patterns and the beauty you are creating.

→ Be aware of your thoughts without reacting to them. As you color these symbols of the harvest, think about the amazing bounty and abundance most Americans enjoy.

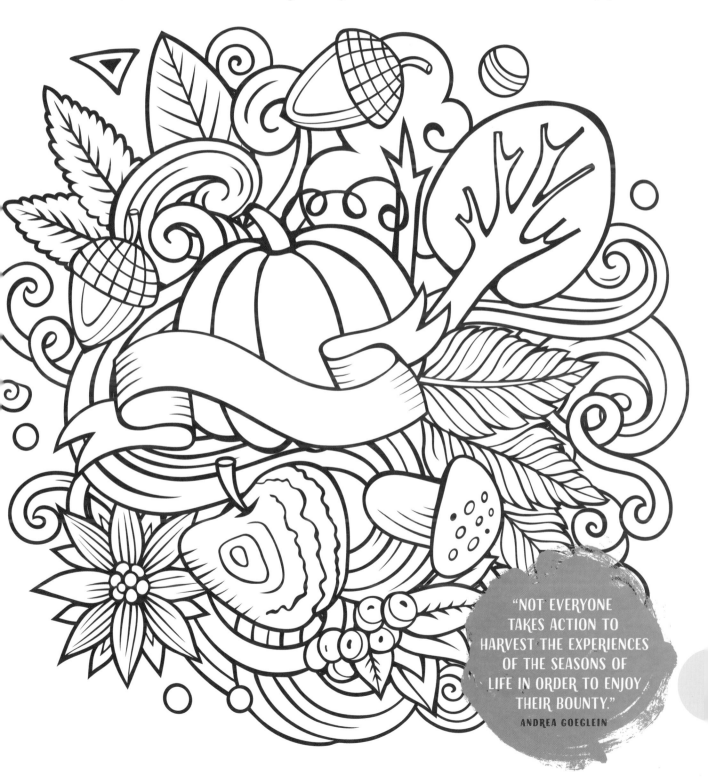

"NOT EVERYONE TAKES ACTION TO HARVEST THE EXPERIENCES OF THE SEASONS OF LIFE IN ORDER TO ENJOY THEIR BOUNTY."

ANDREA GOEGLEIN

Record your activities and thoughts for every day of the week.

S

M

T

W

T

F

S

🌷 TO-DO LIST

_____

_____

_____

_____

_____

Mood Chart							
	S	M	T	W	T	F	S
☀							
⛅							
☁							
🌦							
🌧							
⛈							

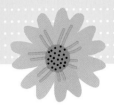

MINDFULNESS TOOLBOX JOURNALING EXERCISE

List 10 things that we take for granted that are not available to many
other people in the world (i.e. clean running water, ample food, electricity).

1

2

3

4

5

6

7

8

9

10

"NO ONE
EVER SOWED THE
GRAIN OF GENEROSITY
WHO GATHERED NOT
UP THE HARVEST
OF THE DESIRE OF
HIS HEART."
SAADI

Record your activities and thoughts for every day of the week.

S

M

T

W

T

F

S

🌷 TO-DO LIST

_____

_____

_____

_____

_____

Mood Chart	S	M	T	W	T	F	S
☀							
⛅							
☁							
🌧							
⛆							
⛈							

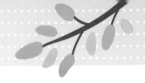

MINDFULNESS TOOLBOX JOURNALING EXERCISE

Write a personal ad for yourself.

What are your likes, your dislikes; why are other people attracted to you?

"LOVE IS
COMPOSED OF
A SINGLE SOUL
INHABITING
TWO BODIES."
ARISTOTLE

DECEMBER 11 – DECEMBER 17

Record your activities and thoughts for every day of the week.

S

M

T

W

T

F

S

🪷 TO-DO LIST

_____
_____
_____
_____
_____

Mood Chart

	S	M	T	W	T	F	S
☀️							
⛅							
☁️							
🌧️							
⛈️							
🌩️							

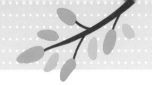

MINDFULNESS TOOLBOX RELAXATION EXERCISE

STOP is a practice developed by mindfulness-based stress reduction (MBSR) founder Jon Kabat-Zinn, PhD. Each letter represents a step to take when you're feeling stressed or overwhelmed.

→ **Stop and pause for a moment.**

→ **Take a breath.**

→ **Observe and acknowledge what is happening.**

→ **Proceed; having briefly checked in with the present moment, you're in a better state of mind to continue with whatever it was you were doing.**

When did you use this technique this week?

Was it helpful?

When do you think it might be helpful?

> "THE GREATEST WEAPON AGAINST STRESS IS OUR ABILITY TO CHOOSE ONE THOUGHT OVER ANOTHER."
> **WILLIAM JAMES**

DECEMBER 18 – DECEMBER 24

Record your activities and thoughts for every day of the week.

S

M FIRST DAY OF HANUKKAH

T

W FIRST DAY OF WINTER

T

F

S

❀ TO-DO LIST

_____

_____

_____

_____

Mood Chart

	S	M	T	W	T	F	S
☀							
⛅							
☁							
🌧							
🌧							
⛈							

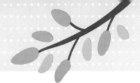

MINDFULNESS TOOLBOX JOURNALING EXERCISE

What was your favorite holiday season ever?
Describe it—how old were you, where were you, who else was there?

_____

_____

_____

_____

_____

_____

What made it so special?

_____

_____

_____

_____

_____

_____

What aspect of that would you like to capture
this holiday season?

_____

_____

_____

_____

_____

"OUR HEARTS GROW
TENDER WITH CHILDHOOD
MEMORIES AND LOVE
OF KINDRED, AND WE ARE
BETTER THROUGHOUT THE
YEAR FOR HAVING, IN SPIRIT,
BECOME A CHILD AGAIN
AT CHRISTMAS-TIME."

LAURA INGALLS WILDER

Record your activities and thoughts for every day of the week.

S CHRISTMAS DAY

M FIRST DAY OF KWANZAA

T

W

T

F

S

🌷 TO-DO LIST

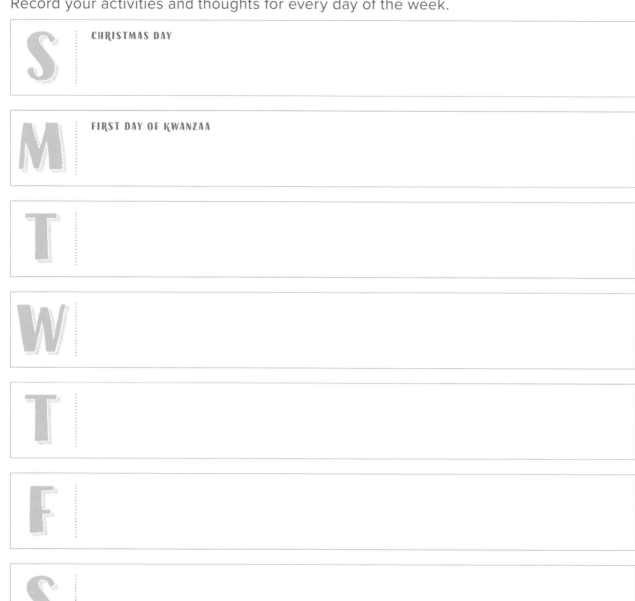

Mood Chart	S	M	T	W	T	F	S
☀							
⛅							
☁							
🌧							
🌧							
⛈							

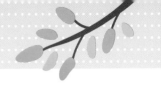

MINDFULNESS TOOLBOX COLORING EXERCISE

To make coloring mindful, follow these guidelines:

→ Set aside 15 minutes when you won't be interrupted.

→ Don't try to focus on anything specific; just pay attention to the colors, the patterns and the beauty you are creating.

→ Be aware of your thoughts without reacting to them. As you color these presents, think about the joy you'll have in giving gifts this holiday season.

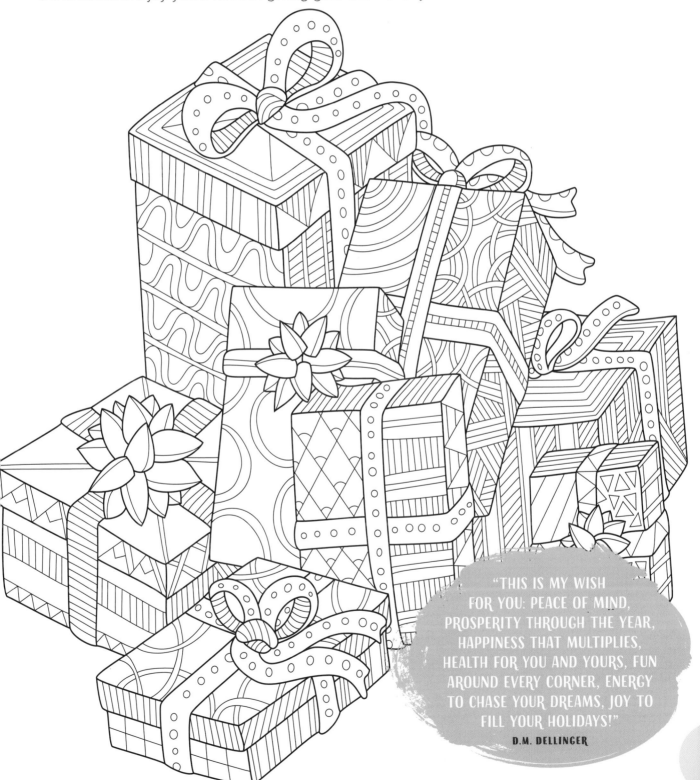

"THIS IS MY WISH FOR YOU: PEACE OF MIND, PROSPERITY THROUGH THE YEAR, HAPPINESS THAT MULTIPLIES, HEALTH FOR YOU AND YOURS, FUN AROUND EVERY CORNER, ENERGY TO CHASE YOUR DREAMS, JOY TO FILL YOUR HOLIDAYS!"

D.M. DELLINGER

NOTES

"EACH NEW DAY IS A BLANK PAGE IN THE DIARY OF YOUR LIFE. THE SECRET OF SUCCESS IS IN TURNING THAT DIARY INTO THE BEST STORY YOU POSSIBLY CAN."
DOUGLAS PAGELS

Special Thanks to Contributing Writers
Amanda Altman · Hallie Levine
All art by **Shutterstock**

CENTENNIAL BOOKS

An Imprint of
Centennial Media, LLC
1111 Brickell Avenue, 10th Floor
Miami, FL 33131, U.S.A.

CENTENNIAL BOOKS is a trademark of Centennial Media, LLC

ISBN 978-1-951274-88-7

Distributed by
Simon & Schuster, Inc.
1230 Avenue of the Americas
New York, NY 10020, U.S.A.

For information about custom editions, special sales and premium and corporate purchases, please contact Centennial Media at contact@centennialmedia.com.

Manufactured in China

10 9 8 7 6 5 4 3 2 1

Publishers & Co-Founders Ben Harris, Sebastian Raatz
Editorial Director Annabel Vered
Creative Director Jessica Power
Executive Editor Janet Giovanelli
Features Editor Alyssa Shaffer
Deputy Editor Ron Kelly
Managing Editor Lisa Chambers
Design Director Martin Elfers
Senior Art Director Pino Impastato
Art Directors Jaclyn Loney, Natali Suasnavas, Joseph Ulatowski
Copy/Production Patty Carroll, Angela Taormina
Senior Photo Editor Jenny Veiga
Production Manager Paul Rodina
Production Assistant Alyssa Swiderski
Editorial Assistant Tiana Schippa
Sales & Marketing Jeremy Nurnberg